MY NAME

&

MY GOAL

DATE: _____

Breakfast:
_____
_____
_____
_____
_____

Lunch:
_____
_____
_____
_____
_____

Dinner:
_____
_____
_____
_____
_____
_____
_____

Snacks:
_____
_____
_____
_____

Exercise/Activity:

Cravings/Response:

Sleep : _____. Hours.

Water Intake:

How I Feel:

It will be better tomorrow:

DATE:_____

Breakfast:

Lunch:

Dinner:

Snacks:

Exercise/Activity:

Cravings/Response:

Sleep : _____ Hours.

Water Intake:

How I Feel:

It will be better tomorrow:

DATE:_____

Breakfast:

Lunch:

Dinner:

Snacks:

Exercise/Activity:

Cravings/Response:

Sleep : _____ Hours.

Water Intake:

How I Feel:

It will be better tomorrow:

DATE:_____

Breakfast:

Lunch:

Dinner:

Snacks:

Exercise/Activity:

Cravings/Response:

Sleep : _____ Hours.

Water Intake:

How I Feel:

It will be better tomorrow:

DATE:_____

Breakfast:

Lunch:

Dinner:

Snacks:

Exercise/Activity:
_____
_____
_____

Cravings/Response:
_____
_____
_____

Sleep : _____ Hours.

Water Intake:

How I Feel:
_____
_____

😀 🙂 😐 ☹️

It will be better tomorrow:
_____
_____
_____

DATE: _____

Breakfast:
_____
_____
_____
_____

Lunch:
_____
_____
_____
_____

Dinner:
_____
_____
_____
_____
_____
_____

Snacks:
_____
_____
_____
_____

Exercise/Activity:
_____
_____
_____

Cravings/Response:
_____
_____
_____

Sleep : _____ Hours.

Water Intake:

⊔⊔⊔⊔⊔⊔⊔⊔⊔

How I Feel:
_____
_____

😀 🙂 😐 🙁

It will be better tomorrow:
_____
_____
_____

DATE:_____

Breakfast:

Lunch:

Dinner:

Snacks:

Exercise/Activity:

Cravings/Response:

Sleep : _____ Hours.

Water Intake:

How I Feel:

It will be better tomorrow:

DATE:_____

Breakfast:

Lunch:

Dinner:

Snacks:

Exercise/Activity:

Cravings/Response:

Sleep : _____ Hours.

Water Intake:

How I Feel:

It will be better tomorrow:

DATE:_____

Breakfast:

Lunch:

Dinner:

Snacks:

Exercise/Activity:
_____
_____

Cravings/Response:
_____
_____

Sleep : _____ Hours.

Water Intake:

How I Feel:
_____
_____

😀 🙂 😐 ☹️

It will be better tomorrow:
_____
_____

DATE:_____

Breakfast:

Lunch:

Dinner:

Snacks:

Exercise/Activity:

Cravings/Response:

Sleep : _____ Hours.

Water Intake:

How I Feel:

It will be better tomorrow:

DATE: _____

Breakfast:

Lunch:

Dinner:

Snacks:

Exercise/Activity:
_____
_____
_____

Cravings/Response:
_____
_____
_____

Sleep : _____ Hours.

Water Intake:

How I Feel:
_____
_____

😀 🙂 😐 🙁

It will be better tomorrow:
_____
_____
_____

DATE:_____

Breakfast:

Lunch:

Dinner:

Snacks:

Exercise/Activity:

Cravings/Response:

Sleep : _____ Hours.

Water Intake:

How I Feel:

It will be better tomorrow:

DATE:_____

Breakfast:

Lunch:

Dinner:

Snacks:

Exercise/Activity:

Cravings/Response:

Sleep : _____. Hours.

Water Intake:

How I Feel:

It will be better tomorrow:

DATE:_____

Breakfast:

Lunch:

Dinner:

Snacks:

Exercise/Activity:

Cravings/Response:

Sleep : _____. Hours.

Water Intake:

How I Feel:

It will be better tomorrow:

DATE:_____

Breakfast:

Lunch:

Dinner:

Snacks:

Exercise/Activity:
_____
_____
_____

Cravings/Response:
_____
_____
_____

Sleep : _____ Hours.

Water Intake:

🥛🥛🥛🥛🥛🥛🥛🥛🥛

How I Feel:
_____
_____

😃 🙂 😐 ☹️

It will be better tomorrow:
_____
_____
_____

DATE: _____

Breakfast:
_____
_____
_____
_____

Lunch:
_____
_____
_____
_____

Dinner:
_____
_____
_____
_____
_____

Snacks:
_____
_____
_____
_____

Exercise/Activity:
_____
_____
_____

Cravings/Response:
_____
_____
_____

Sleep : _____ Hours.

Water Intake:

How I Feel:
_____
_____

It will be better tomorrow:
_____
_____
_____

DATE:_____

Breakfast:

Lunch:

Dinner:

Snacks:

Exercise/Activity:

Cravings/Response:

Sleep : _____. Hours.

Water Intake:

How I Feel:

It will be better tomorrow:

DATE: _____

Breakfast:

Lunch:

Dinner:

Snacks:

Exercise/Activity:

Cravings/Response:

Sleep : _____ Hours.

Water Intake:

How I Feel:

It will be better tomorrow:

DATE:_____

Breakfast:

Lunch:

Dinner:

Snacks:

Exercise/Activity:

Cravings/Response:

Sleep : _____. Hours.

Water Intake:

How I Feel:

It will be better tomorrow:

DATE:_____

Breakfast:

Lunch:

Dinner:

Snacks:

Exercise/Activity:

Cravings/Response:

Sleep : _____ Hours.

Water Intake:

How I Feel:

It will be better tomorrow:

DATE: _____

Breakfast:

_____
_____
_____
_____

Lunch:

_____
_____
_____
_____

Dinner:

_____
_____
_____
_____
_____
_____

Snacks:

_____
_____
_____
_____

Exercise/Activity:

Cravings/Response:

Sleep : _____ Hours.

Water Intake:

How I Feel:

It will be better tomorrow:

DATE: _____

Breakfast:

Lunch:

Dinner:

Snacks:

Exercise/Activity:

Cravings/Response:

Sleep : _____ Hours.

Water Intake:

How I Feel:

It will be better tomorrow:

DATE:_____

Breakfast:

Lunch:

Dinner:

Snacks:

Exercise/Activity:

Cravings/Response:

Sleep : _____ Hours.

Water Intake:

How I Feel:

It will be better tomorrow:

DATE:_____

Breakfast:
_____
_____
_____
_____

Lunch:
_____
_____
_____
_____

Dinner:
_____
_____
_____
_____
_____
_____

Snacks:
_____
_____
_____
_____

Exercise/Activity:

Cravings/Response:

Sleep : _____ Hours.

Water Intake:

How I Feel:

It will be better tomorrow:

DATE: _____

Breakfast:
_____
_____
_____
_____
_____

Lunch:
_____
_____
_____
_____
_____

Dinner:
_____
_____
_____
_____
_____
_____

Snacks:
_____
_____
_____
_____

Exercise/Activity:
_____
_____
_____

Cravings/Response:
_____
_____
_____

Sleep : _____ Hours.

Water Intake:

How I Feel:
_____
_____

It will be better tomorrow:
_____
_____
_____

DATE:_____

Breakfast:

Lunch:

Dinner:

Snacks:

Exercise/Activity:

Cravings/Response:

Sleep : _____ Hours.

Water Intake:

How I Feel:

It will be better tomorrow:

DATE:_____

Breakfast:

Lunch:

Dinner:

Snacks:

Exercise/Activity:

Cravings/Response:

Sleep : _____ Hours.

Water Intake:

How I Feel:

It will be better tomorrow:

DATE:_____

Breakfast:

Lunch:

Dinner:

Snacks:

Exercise/Activity:
_____
_____
_____

Cravings/Response:
_____
_____
_____

Sleep : _____ Hours.

Water Intake:

How I Feel:
_____
_____
_____

😃 🙂 😐 ☹️

It will be better tomorrow:
_____
_____
_____

DATE:_____

Breakfast:

Lunch:

Dinner:

Snacks:

Exercise/Activity:

Cravings/Response:

Sleep : _____. Hours.

Water Intake:

How I Feel:

It will be better tomorrow:

DATE: _____

Breakfast:
_____
_____
_____
_____
_____

Lunch:
_____
_____
_____
_____
_____

Dinner:
_____
_____
_____
_____
_____
_____

Snacks:
_____
_____
_____
_____

Exercise/Activity:

Cravings/Response:

Sleep : _____ Hours.

Water Intake:

How I Feel:

It will be better tomorrow:

DATE:_____

Breakfast:

Lunch:

Dinner:

Snacks:

Exercise/Activity:
_____
_____

Cravings/Response:
_____
_____

Sleep : _____. Hours.

Water Intake:

How I Feel:
_____
_____

It will be better tomorrow:
_____
_____
_____

DATE:_____

Breakfast:
_____
....
....
_____

Lunch:
_____
....
....
....
_____

Dinner:
_____
....
....
....
....
....
_____

Snacks:
_____
....
....
....
_____

Exercise/Activity:
_____
_____
_____

Cravings/Response:
_____
_____
_____

Sleep : _____ Hours.

Water Intake:

How I Feel:
_____
_____
_____

It will be better tomorrow:
_____
_____
_____

DATE:_____

Breakfast:

Lunch:

Dinner:

Snacks:

Exercise/Activity:

Cravings/Response:

Sleep : _____ Hours.

Water Intake:

How I Feel:

It will be better tomorrow:

DATE: _____

Breakfast:
....
....
....
....

Lunch:
....
....
....
....

Dinner:
....
....
....
....
....
....

Snacks:
....
....
....
....

Exercise/Activity:

Cravings/Response:

Sleep : _____. Hours.

Water Intake:

How I Feel:

It will be better tomorrow:

DATE:_____

Breakfast:

Lunch:

Dinner:

Snacks:

Exercise/Activity:

Cravings/Response:

Sleep : _____ Hours.

Water Intake:

How I Feel:

It will be better tomorrow:

DATE: _____

Breakfast:
_____
_____
_____
_____

Lunch:
_____
_____
_____
_____

Dinner:
_____
_____
_____
_____
_____
_____

Snacks:
_____
_____
_____
_____

Exercise/Activity:

Cravings/Response:

Sleep : _____ Hours.

Water Intake:

How I Feel:

It will be better tomorrow:

DATE: _____

Breakfast:
_____
_____
_____
_____
_____

Lunch:
_____
_____
_____
_____
_____

Dinner:
_____
_____
_____
_____
_____

Snacks:
_____
_____
_____
_____

Exercise/Activity:

Cravings/Response:

Sleep : _____ Hours.

Water Intake:

How I Feel:

It will be better tomorrow:

DATE:_____

Breakfast:

Lunch:

Dinner:

Snacks:

Exercise/Activity:

Cravings/Response:

Sleep : _____ Hours.

Water Intake:

How I Feel:

It will be better tomorrow:

DATE:_____

Breakfast:

Lunch:

Dinner:

Snacks:

Exercise/Activity:
_____
_____
_____

Cravings/Response:
_____
_____
_____

Sleep : _____ Hours.

Water Intake:

How I Feel:
_____

😀 🙂 😐 🙁

It will be better tomorrow:
_____
_____
_____

DATE:_____

Breakfast:

Lunch:

Dinner:

Snacks:

Exercise/Activity:
_____
_____
_____

Cravings/Response:
_____
_____
_____

Sleep : _____ Hours.

Water Intake:

How I Feel:
_____
_____

It will be better tomorrow:
_____
_____
_____

DATE:_____

Breakfast:
_____
_____
_____
_____

Lunch:
_____
_____
_____
_____

Dinner:
_____
_____
_____
_____
_____
_____

Snacks:
_____
_____
_____
_____

Exercise/Activity:

Cravings/Response:

Sleep : _____ Hours.

Water Intake:

How I Feel:

It will be better tomorrow:

DATE: _____

Breakfast:

_____
_____
_____
_____

Lunch:

_____
_____
_____
_____
_____

Dinner:

_____
_____
_____
_____
_____
_____
_____

Snacks:

_____
_____
_____
_____

Exercise/Activity:

Cravings/Response:

Sleep : _____ Hours.

Water Intake:

How I Feel:

It will be better tomorrow:

DATE:_____

Breakfast:

Lunch:

Dinner:

Snacks:

Exercise/Activity:

Cravings/Response:

Sleep : _____ Hours.

Water Intake:

How I Feel:

It will be better tomorrow:

DATE: _____

Breakfast:

Lunch:

Dinner:

Snacks:

Exercise/Activity:
_____
_____

Cravings/Response:
_____
_____

Sleep : _____ Hours.

Water Intake:

How I Feel:
_____
_____

😀 🙂 😐 🙁

It will be better tomorrow:
_____
_____

DATE:_____

Breakfast:

Lunch:

Dinner:

Snacks:

Exercise/Activity:
_____
_____

Cravings/Response:
_____
_____
_____

Sleep : _____ Hours.

Water Intake:

How I Feel:
_____
_____

😃 🙂 😐 ☹️

It will be better tomorrow:
_____
_____
_____

DATE: _____

Breakfast:

Lunch:

Dinner:

Snacks:

Exercise/Activity:
_____
_____
_____

Cravings/Response:
_____
_____
_____

Sleep : _____ Hours.

Water Intake:

How I Feel:
_____
_____

It will be better tomorrow:
_____
_____
_____

DATE:_____

Breakfast:

Lunch:

Dinner:

Snacks:

Exercise/Activity:

Cravings/Response:

Sleep : _____. Hours.

Water Intake:

How I Feel:

It will be better tomorrow:

DATE:_____

Breakfast:

Lunch:

Dinner:

Snacks:

Exercise/Activity:

Cravings/Response:

Sleep : _____ Hours.

Water Intake:

How I Feel:

It will be better tomorrow:

DATE: _____

Breakfast:

_____
_____
_____
_____

Lunch:

_____
_____
_____
_____

Dinner:

_____
_____
_____
_____
_____
_____

Snacks:

_____
_____
_____
_____

Exercise/Activity:

Cravings/Response:

Sleep : _____. Hours.

Water Intake:

How I Feel:

It will be better tomorrow:

DATE: _____

Breakfast:

Lunch:

Dinner:

Snacks:

Exercise/Activity:

Cravings/Response:

Sleep : _____ Hours.

Water Intake:

How I Feel:

It will be better tomorrow:

DATE:_____

Breakfast:

Lunch:

Dinner:

Snacks:

Exercise/Activity:

Cravings/Response:

Sleep : _____ Hours.

Water Intake:

How I Feel:

It will be better tomorrow:

DATE:_____

Breakfast:

Lunch:

Dinner:

Snacks:

Exercise/Activity:

Cravings/Response:

Sleep : _____ Hours.

Water Intake:

How I Feel:

It will be better tomorrow:

DATE:_____

Breakfast:

Lunch:

Dinner:

Snacks:

Exercise/Activity:

Cravings/Response:

Sleep : _____. Hours.

Water Intake:

How I Feel:

It will be better tomorrow:

DATE:_____

Breakfast:

_____
_____
_____
_____

Lunch:

_____
_____
_____
_____

Dinner:

_____
_____
_____
_____
_____
_____

Snacks:

_____
_____
_____
_____

Exercise/Activity:

Cravings/Response:

Sleep : _____. Hours.

Water Intake:

How I Feel:

It will be better tomorrow:

DATE: _____

Breakfast:

Lunch:

Dinner:

Snacks:

Exercise/Activity:

Cravings/Response:

Sleep : _____. Hours.

Water Intake:

How I Feel:

It will be better tomorrow:

DATE:_____

Breakfast:

Lunch:

Dinner:

Snacks:

Exercise/Activity:

Cravings/Response:

Sleep : _____. Hours.

Water Intake:

How I Feel:

It will be better tomorrow:

DATE:_____

Breakfast:

_____
_____
_____
_____

Lunch:

_____
_____
_____
_____

Dinner:

_____
_____
_____
_____
_____
_____

Snacks:

_____
_____
_____
_____

Exercise/Activity:

Cravings/Response:

Sleep : _____ Hours.

Water Intake:

How I Feel:

It will be better tomorrow:

DATE: _____

Breakfast:

Lunch:

Dinner:

Snacks:

Exercise/Activity:
_____
_____

Cravings/Response:
_____
_____

Sleep : _____. Hours.

Water Intake:

How I Feel:
_____
_____

It will be better tomorrow:
_____
_____
_____

DATE:_____

Breakfast:

Lunch:

Dinner:

Snacks:

Exercise/Activity:
_____
_____
_____

Cravings/Response:
_____
_____
_____

Sleep : _____. Hours.

Water Intake:

How I Feel:
_____
_____
_____

It will be better tomorrow:
_____
_____
_____

DATE: _____

Breakfast:

Lunch:

Dinner:

Snacks:

Exercise/Activity:

Cravings/Response:

Sleep : _____. Hours.

Water Intake:

How I Feel:

It will be better tomorrow:

www.ingramcontent.com/pod-product-compliance
Lightning Source LLC
Chambersburg PA
CBHW050312230526
45471CB00005B/2135